Your Natural Health Revolution
Going from S.A.D. to G.L.A.D.

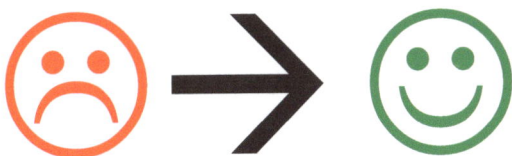

Table of Contents

This book is dedicated to the Creator who's name is YAHWEH the ELohim of YisraEL!

Yael YisraEL would like to dedicate this book to Emma and Abba(May YAH be with your Spirit Abba) Who've always showed me to live healthy and true!

I.M. YisraEL & Yael would like to also dedicate this book to our children, for YAH desires that man and woman shall be one so that we may raise a Holy Seed!

Part I: Introduction To Natural Living

The current state of health care and nutrition today is one of drastic confusion and oversaturated marketing schemes to influence you to by artificial products erroneously called food and medicine. Further more we are being victimized by murders, thieves, and con artist who call themselves; doctors, scientist, and health professionals. If you would like to be healthy enjoy life and have long life then we invite you to partake in the new revolution, your natural health revolution!

Now some of you might be thinking; "I already eat natural I'm a vegetarian, I eat eggs, fish, cheese and take vitamins, herbs, and homeopathic medication. I get regular colonics and eat beans and brown rice." If you have thought the previous quote or any part of it then you are not living a natural lifestyle. What we are going to do is break down the basics of Modern medical health care and nutrition, Alternative heath care and nutrition, and reveal what really is Natural health care and nutrition. We will do this with out romantically meandering about the view points of the high polluted so-called doctors, and health masters, and gurus.

The Doctors

First things first: Modern Health Science- I call this culture of health care and nutrition modern health science because it is the contemporary thought or what health is based on modern science.

Science at it's very nature is the wrong field to dictate what is and what isn't healthy for us simply because, modern science does not acknowledge the creator nor believe everything the creator has made is perfect.

Science has given the public a food guide that leads you to a doctor's office. They used to show a pyramid but now there is a plate and the easiest way for us to understand what science wants us eat is to simply look at the plate:

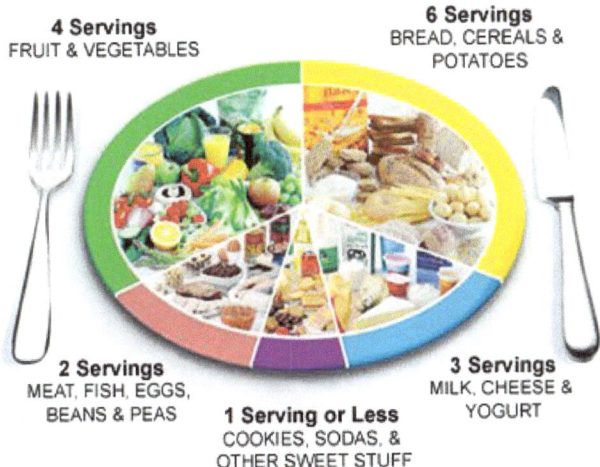

4 Servings
FRUIT & VEGETABLES

6 Servings
BREAD, CEREALS &
POTATOES

2 Servings
MEAT, FISH, EGGS,
BEANS & PEAS

1 Serving or Less
COOKIES, SODAS, &
OTHER SWEET STUFF

3 Servings
MILK, CHEESE &
YOGURT

By looking at the new recommendations of how we should eat, we see that the scientists would like to kill us.

First indication that they would like us to die slowly is that they suggested we eat 3 whooping servings of Milk, Cheese, and Yogurt.

Milk creates mucus in our bodies starves us of oxygen. Cheese and yogurt does the same.

Then the *smart ones* tell us to eat 2 servings of Meat, fish (fish is meat), Beans, eggs, and peas. Eating Meat 2x's a day is horribly excessive, and is outright poison when speaking of the meat purchased in the stores today. This toxic meat will never and has never given our bodies oxygen, help increase our energy, and meat can not increase circulation. These three activities are essential to maintain a healthy body, heart, and spirit.

6 servings of dead grain are what they want you to consume, and/or potatoes. This is all starch and will turn into sugar, and mucus. Again starving our bodies of the three essential actions.

1 serving of cookies, sodas, or sweet stuff! LOL! You already know this is evil, and outright wickedness, never should you eat just any sweet stuff, you should never drink soda or fruit juice with out the bubbles. Cookies or any other product made with any processed sugar: brown, cane, turbinatto, raw, processed stevia, etc. is hell to your blood stream.

Finally 4 servings of fruits and vegetables, the entire plate should be fruits, vegetables, and water there is no section for water... I can't believe it!

When it comes to doctor visits, and medicine, this as we should realize by now is a factory of murder. Allopathic medicine does not believe in letting the body heal it's self. Instead, allopathic medicine believes the body is helpless and needs to be fooled into thinking that the pain and symptoms are gone. All medications hide symptoms, all surgeries eliminate an isolated "problem." If I'm in pain, they'll give me a pain killer, but it will not heal the cause of the pain, pain is just a indicator to a problem not the problem itself. If I cannot loose weight, they'll sew my stomach, if my heart is failing they'll bypass the clogged artery. If my leg won't heal, they'll cut it off and so on and so forth. This method of medical treatment is not healing, it is not healthy and it is not natural at all.

All sickness that we adopt in our bodies, are due to what we put in us. There is not a disease that one has that does not have its root in our diet or environment. That being said, the extra smart M.D.'s should know this... right? Wrong! The MD'S know nothing of nutrition. Do not ever expect a doctor to give you a prescription for herbs, or natural supplements, they would not know where to begin.

The super smart doctors are trained to think that genetics, and unfortunate birthing defects are the culprits behind illness. They feel they can out smart nature and that nature made a sh!@ load of genetic mistakes, and now the doctors have to figure out how to fix our genetics; hence the Human Genome Project. **"The ultimate goal of this initiative is to understand the human genome" and "knowledge of the human is as necessary to the continuing progress of medicine and other health sciences as knowledge of human anatomy has been for the present state of medicine." (Wikipedia.org)**

The scientist can have their genome map and will never learn how to cure cancer, aids, malaria, or the common cold, because even genetics are subordinate to what we put in our bodies.

Is It Really Holistic Health?

Moving on to the now glossy alternative or so-called holistic health. There are many methods to healing and health, therefore we will not dissect each one, and we will examine the most popular methods.

We have already commented on Allopathic medicine briefly we will now go to what is called "Holistic Health." In holistic health we have been led to believe that it is a natural method to living and healing. Yes, holistic health focuses on natural methods, but holistic health is not innately natural.

Lets' look at Homeopathy for instance: Homeopathy means: the treatment of disease by minute doses of natural substances that in a healthy person would produce symptoms of disease. Often contrasted with **allopath** . Now we can see from this definition that homeopathy is not absolutely natural. Homeopathy does consider diet, environment, mental state and the other causes of dis-ease, but it does not treat dis-ease naturally. Like allopathic medicine homeopathy attempts to force the body to heal itself. Vaccinations force the body to create immunities to a certain infection, this in theory will cause the body to fight off these "viruses." In homeopathic medicine homeopaths administer poisonous plants greatly diluted to cause the body to heal one's self. This process does work but it is not perfect, and it is not natural, therefore it is not true health, homeopathic medication I would recommend very rarely, if at all.

Next we have Herbalists, Naturopathic Doctors, Reki, Iridologist, Chakra coaches, Holistic Nutritionist, etc, etc. The list of isolated specialist in the realm of holistic health is about as abundant as the specialist in allopathic health. The one thing all these specialist have in common is that none of them are 100% natural. The reason for the unnatural health care in a naturally founded method is because of money, and ignorance. When I became a professional Herbalist, I was taught like everyone else that soy, beans, potatoes, carrots, garlic, apple cider vinegar, oranges, and collard greens were natural and good food to eat. One thing my instructor taught me which resounded over and over was; natural means that it has grown on it own with no help or assistance from man. Therefore when we look at what a common herbalist might recommend for you, it might be a plant or plant based supplement, but it won't always be a natural plant. Then holistic practices support allopathic health care by recommending x-rays, MRI, biopsies, or allopathic treatment for trauma. Ask yourself, in the ancient times, or in the indigenous societies, where vicodin or valium is not available for immediate pain relief, and a defibrillator, what did they or what do they do to preserve life and ease excruciating pain? The answer is herbs. Natural herbs, can and will stop heart attacks, strokes, seizures, relieve tremendous pain, fix broken bones, stop bleeding, heal wombs, return people from comas, prevent mis-carriages, break fevers, dissolve tumors, and so on and so forth. So why do naturopaths recommend allopathic treatment for these situations? They do it because they do not know how to treat them or they are to afraid of the herbs not working.

The diet that most naturopaths recommend for people to partake in is not natural at all, nor are the herbs they recommend natural and some of the food they'll attempt to sell you is down right death in a leaf. Let me explain what is natural and what is not natural.

What Is Natural?

The Creator of the Heaven, earth, sea , and universe who's name is YAH, made all things and the vegetation he made all, I repeat **ALL** have seeds. Therefore when we start consuming items with no seeds then we are dealing with an un-natural food. These items cause health risks, because they are all more acidic than their natural parent, most fruits and vegetables are alkaline or will turn alkaline when they enter into your body. Then the Creator again let us know that we should not sow our field with mingled seed because this will defile the fruit or our gardens. Monsanto, and DuPont just to name a couple are mingling plant seeds all over America and trying to get the world hooked on GMO food. Genetically Modified food is mingled not only with other plant seed, but with animal genes, insect genes, *maybe even human genes*, just to create a greater yield of the product in order to make gross amounts of money.

Some foods that have been mingled from thousands of years ago are; oranges, garlic, lemons, rice. These foods have been mingled with different fruit and vegetable seeds for variety and taste. Garlic is a poison that will not only kill bacteria, it will kill the host of the bacteria. You can liken garlic to fire. If you put fire in your veins you will kill bacteria and the vein, and this is the same process with garlic. The PH of Garlic is 3, and garlic was used in WWI, soldiers would put garlic on their bayonets and stab their enemy poisoning them to death! With Garlic! Living and eating natural is not a gravely challenging task, unless you've been living and eating unnatural for most of your life. I've witnessed with my son, which was blessed to be born at a time when my family was transitioning to a more natural way of eating. This little YAH seed has not had the unfortunate experience of being raised on garbage, but has had a 90% completely natural diet. As a result he does not like any unnatural food naturally!

As adults it is very difficult to get into the grove of eating and living natural. We should start with knowing why foods that are natural are much better for you. If you take a gander at a package of Black rice, Quinoa, Spelt, and Rye you will see that they are all marketed as a SUPER food, and they'll say that these foods are complete proteins. The reason for this is because these grains are Natural and they have all the minerals that the ground gives them. By having a complete mineral distribution in your natural foods, this phrase *complete protein* is automatic. In addition you now have a food marketed as SUPER!

Unnatural foods have to be enriched. White rice, brown rice, orange juice, milk, cheese, wheat bread and wheat products will all be marketed as enriched... This is because they have been depleted. Processed foods are unnatural. Recommendations from doctors and herbalist alike for a completely nutritious meal will sound like this: Eat brown rice, and some seeds and beans with a green vegetable and another "protein" product. This is recommended because the brown rice is a incomplete food, along with the beans and most cases the seeds, the greens will probably be your only complete food if it is not processed. The pseudo health professionals do not know that if you just ate Wild or Black rice, Quinoa, Kale or other natural foods you wouldn't have to worry about getting a *balanced meal* because all your food is natural, and a false balance is a abomination to YAH, therefore none of his natural foods are imbalanced.

Have you ever wondered why we see people who claim they are vegetarians have gained more weight? This is because the unnatural food eaten by vegetarians. Corn is starch, white, brown and golden Rice are starches, Beans are starch, Potatoes are starch, Noodles are starch, Soy, and Seitan are starch. These aforementioned foods are staples not only in a vegetarian diet but also in most humans diet period. What this starch does is cause not only mucus build up but also sugar which turns into fat and then you have a fat starch eating chemicaltarian, because none of these foods aforementioned are real and they are all results of laboratories and chemicals.

The Most High did not make white rice, or white potatoes, white wheat or wheat period, white or yellow corn, white beans, white noodles, and white spongy substances called soy and seitan. Therefore if you are planning to become a vegan or vegetarian it would behoove you to not start out like I and so many others have eating these foods and becoming addicted to them, but start out on the right foot, and eat the natural foods that are made from the earth. The process is simple, when you decide to go shopping do your research and see if the food you are about to eat was made in a lab or from the beginning of time with seeds and all supplying our souls with minerals. If this is not the case the food is not natural and will do your body more harm that good.

Part II
Going From S.A.D. To G.L.A.D.

S.A.D. The Standard American Diet, is truly a sad state. The Standard American Diet you can find on the plate in part I of this book. The SAD eating habits is more than just eating sad, but it is also living sad. You are what you eat. If one is eating bacon, shrimp, drinking soda pop, eating fried foods, smoking, drinking alcohol, taking illegal or prescription drugs, than your on a level of living the S.A.D. Life.

What we have to do is revolutionize our eating habits. The first steps to changing our eating habits is to fortify a mental standard that you will not continue to poison your self, because you love your self and want to live life to the best of your ability! We have to enjoy life, and pain and pesky colds, allergies, looming cancers, and other diseases are not helping us enjoy life. These aforementioned diseases are a consequence of the S.A.D. lifestyle.

Therefore how do we embark on this revolution? As already stated; get your mind right first. Next we have to know what we should be eating and what we should not be eating. Here is a list of foods we should not eat:

- Beans
- Corn

- White, Brown, Patty, Golden, Basmati, or Jasmine Rice
- White Potatoes
- White Flour (Wheat),
- Wheat
- White Sugar, Brown Sugar, Molasses, Raw Sugar, Aspartame
- Collard Greens
- Soy
- Oranges
- Garlic
- Bananas
- Pineapples
- Beats
- Carrots
- Sweet Potatoes
- Dairy
- Meat; especially Pork, and shell fish.

WHAT!!! This might be what many of you are saying… Beans are nothing but starch and a highly GMO food, the only beans I recommend are Chick peas, string beans, lentils and split peas. Corn is not for human consumption, in addition to that corn is engineered in a lab and has not been real food since the 1800's. If the rice is not black do not eat it. Rice is Engineered and a starch. All the food on this list is unnatural and acidic, and very dangerous for our bodies and very, very dangerous to give to our children.

"Well, What can I eat?" This is your next question. There are plenty of foods we can eat. Your shopping will definitely be modified. A good place to start to shop is your own back yard, if you have one. Other good places are; Farmers markets, and natural/health local food stores.

"This food is too expensive!" Will be your next thought. Yes natural food is a bit more costly than poison... But it's kinda life and death here...

Now after we move past those particulars, what is it that we should eat?

- Water
- Wild, or Black Rice
- Kammut, Teff, Rye, Spelt, Quinoa (All natural grains take the place of wheat and wheat products).
- Kale, Turnip, Mustard Greens
- Spinach
- String Beans
- Most green organic vegetables
- Apples

- Berries
- Grapes with seeds
- Mandarins
- Melons
- Pears
- Plums
- Limes
- Most fruit is natural just make sure you have seeded fruits.

For complete food guides you can go to www.tamiyminc.com, or www.drsebiproducts.com, or www.rahealing.com , here you can find the same food list with minor variations.

Most of the foods we buy in grocery stores are not natural nor are they real. It is not profitable for stores to have rotting food on their shelves, therefore they have lab made food that last for weeks instead of days. Living food must be eaten expeditiously.

The Global Living African Diet is labeled as such because this type of eating is what the ancestors of the entire human race use to eat. Be it that we all originate from Akubalan (Africa), it would make sense to eat how we ate when we inhabited our homeland. In addition to this, all the food we recommend is 100% natural and alive, made directly from the Creator's mouth. If we eat lively food then we will begin to fell lively. If we eat deadly food will feel deathly; it is that simple.

What are the benefits of eating a 100% natural vegan diet:

- Weight Loss
- No Arthritis
- No headaches
- No Heart Burn
- No Back pain
- No Allergies
- No Colds
- No Flu
- Clear Mind
- Plenty of Energy!
- No Dis-Ease!
- Increased Libido, and fertilization

These are only a few of the effects of a 100% natural vegan and mostly raw diet. Not only will your health issues begin to fade, in addition you will begin to feel young again! Your mood will be happy you will feel lighter, your out look on life will become brighter and you will have more patience. The opposite happens when we eat the S.A.D. food. We are irritable, tired, and gloomy, we have aches and pains, mood swings, headaches, etc. etc.

Now we can not transition to a new living habit with our some recipes! We will give you 5 recipes to get started: ;

G.L.A.D. RECIPES

Recipe#1   **Yummy Vegan Pancakes**

1-serving   20 minutes prep. Time

1T raw cane sugar/ agave (optional)
1/2c Spelt Flour
1/4t Baking soda
1/4t baking powder
1/2c Almond milk
1T coconut oil
Handful of chopped fruit
Sprinkle coconut oil

1.) Sift dry ingredients in a large bowl. 2.) Add milk, oil, and mix 3.) Toss handful of fruit in batter 4.) Heat oiled skillet on medium 5.) Pour

2-4 T batter in sprinkle-oiled skillet and cover
6.) Once the middle of cake bubbles and/or
edges seems stiffened, flip the cake and cover
7.) Repeat and keep all cakes in the oven at 200
degrees F to stay warm.

Recipe#2   **Ruby Red Quinoa Soup**

8-10 servings
30 minutes prep time

1-2 chopped tomatoes
1-1/2 c fine string beans
1c spinach
1 lg. chopped yellow onion
1c red quinoa
2 tomatoes puree
cumin, cayenne, sea salt

rinse quinoa, warm tomato puree and 2-
1/2 c water until slightly soupy consistency,
add veggies, and cook down. Add quinoa. Stir,
Simmer 20 minutes

Recipe#3   **Pea Pesto Pasta**

4-6 Servings   15 minutes prep time

Pesto:
1 (10-ounce) package frozen peas, defrosted/ fresh
1 tsp. minced onion
1/2 cup shredded non-dairy cheese
1 tsp. sea salt, plus extra for seasoning
1/4 tsp. red pepper, plus extra for seasoning
1/3c olive oil

Noodles:
1 (9.5 ounce) package spelt spaghetti, cooked

Pulse together the peas, onion, non-dairy cheese, and 1 teaspoon of salt and 1/4 teaspoon of pepper in a food processor. With the machine running, slowly add the olive oil until well combined, about 1 to 2 minutes. Season with additional salt and pepper. Pour the pesto into a bowl of cooked noodles. Stir well.

Recipe#4   **Raw Kale Wrap**

2-4 Servings
30-60 minutes prep time

1 bushel of raw fresh kale
chopped green onions
1 chopped avocado
1 chopped tomato
sea salt
1 lemon
sprouted wraps/pita bread
raw dressing/chickpea humus

First, place fresh kale in a large bowl or a clean kitchen sink with a stopper on the drain. Gradually, squeeze the juice from the lemon onto the kale and add a few pinches of sea salt. Use clean hands to massage the kale until it begins to feel tender. Add the avocado, tomato, and green onions. Continue to massage and mix the ingredients until the kale mixture is very tender. At this point, the kale leaves will seem

smaller and more condense then before. Spread
your favorite raw dressing or chickpea humus
onto a sprouted wrap or pita bread. Add the
raw kale mixture and fold the bread.

Recipe#5   <u>**Vegan Chocolate B-day Cake**</u>

8-12 servings   30 minutes
prep time

1.) Dry mixture

1 1/4c spelt flour
1c raw cane sugar
1/3c organic raw cocoa
1t baking soda
½ t sea salt

2.) Wet mixture

1c warm water
1t vanilla extract
1/3c coconut oil

1t. apple cider vinegar (optional)

Combine wet and dry mixtures in a large bowl. Pour in pan and bake at 350 degrees. Let cake cool, and then glaze.

3.) Glaze

In a small pot add 1/2c raw cane sugar, 4T Earth balance butter, 2T almond milk, 2T cocoa, 2T vanilla. Bring to boil and frequently stir. Remove from heat constantly stirring for about 5 minutes. Immediately, pour onto cake and add walnuts/sprinkles. Let dry.

Fresh Baby Food Meals

1.) Examine, Sort, and Wash desired fresh produce of fruit or veggies for baby. Make sure to use only the meat of the produce, remove all skin, seeds, etc.

2.) Steam food in a steamer, or cook in a covered pot in a small amount of water until tender. Save cooking water to thin baby food, if you desire.

3.) Place food in blender or food processor and puree, adding water as needed until smooth. Serve baby food.

4.) Store extra baby food into ice cube trays, cover with glad wrap, and freeze.

5.) Once frozen, place cubes into freezer bags, date and store in the freezer. Use within 1 month.

6.) When serving, take out the desired number of cubes, warm inside a container floating in covered pot of hot, boiled water, and serve.

Part of living naturally happy is taking care of your outer beauty, and if you can not eat it do not put it on your skin. Here we will look at Natural ways to deal with your Hair, Skin, and nails.

Natural Beauty

There is a common saying that "beauty is in the eye of the beholder". While this is a great idea an even greater one is the fact that beauty is an extension of your inner health (self). There are many internal factors that represent our external appearance from the physical and spiritual realms.

The final destinations of these factors appear in our hair, skin, and nails. Furthermore, there are many external factors that affect the outer beauty. In order to understand and control the natural beauty that one is born with it is important to be aware of the basics of hair, skin, and nails. The main structural constituent found in all three is keratin, which is a fibrous protein. One must also set realistic beauty goals based on preference. It is also significant to be attentive and in tune with your unique self allowing good judgment to rule in order to achieve your beauty goals.

HAIR

The hair is a beauty attribute that can be most complex to understand. Hair is simply the threadlike strands that grow from the scalp. Scientist state hair that has rooted from the follicle is "dead" because the actual cells no longer divide. In this physical sense hair *is* dead. Yet, the great thing about natural hair is that in a spiritual sense it can be considered "alive". Natural hair can send and receive energy vibes like antennas.

The structure of hair include the following: the cuticle is a shingle-like, transparent, protective layers; the cortex is a bundle of proteins containing lipids, water, minerals and pigmentation; the medulla is a mass of cells, not found in all human hair that might regulate body temperature and protection from the sun. Scientists also state that hair growth has 3 cycles: anagen/growth, catagen/transitional (resting), telogen (shedding).

  Some people believe that natural hair is hard to manage. One must consider the question "What does it mean to manage?" All natural hair is manageable if you understand hair. Natural hair comes in four main textures: kinky, curly, wavy, straight.

The first three textures are actual textures considered afro-textured hair. Depending on your type of hair and beauty goals, there are many ways to manage natural hair. For instance, a beauty goal requires different care and technique to obtain good hair health or maintain length, grow long hair, or all of the above. Another relevance to consider when handling hair is the ph balance.

The natural ph of hair is between 4 and 6. Anything above 6 becomes more alkaline and below 4 is too acidic. It is best to mostly stay within the healthy range for hair care. It is always good to have a basic routine, which is not the same as schedule, for your hair. All hair should be cared for very gently, like a piece of fine fabric. In order to have healthy hair and aid achieving any preferred hair goal the basic hair care require the following: Washing, Conditioning, Moisturizing, Detangling, and Protecting. When caring for natural hair, less is best, and always keep it simple.

Keeping clean hair and most importantly a clean scalp is something to be done on a regular basis. This allows your hair to "breathe". It is not essential to use a lot of different types of products on the hair to care for it. Yet, hair can still receive some build up from products, dirt, and grime. It is also very important to be cautious of the ingredients that you use in your hair. It is best to avoid any chemical use on natural hair.

Some shampoos use sulfates which is a detergent used to lather and clean hair stripping it of its natural oils. There are also great techniques to gently clean hair. For example washing hair in sections or in braids can minimize the dangles cause by tousling hair. Using a ph balanced shampoo can support good hair health. Washing in warm temperature water allows the cuticle of the hair strands to lift and be properly cleansed by the water.

Conditioning is a good healthy hair care treatment to implement in a routine. A question to consider when doing this is "What am I conditioning my hair to do?" Depending on your goals and preferences, the two main things that the hair mainly need to be conditioned to do is maintain moisture and be strong. Moisture comes from water and strong hair from something called protein, which is a natural component of hair. It is vital to maintain a healthy balance of moisture and strength for natural hair to thrive. Most afro-textured hair may want to use moisture-rich conditioners in the hair regularly because the hair has a tendency to be dry. The hair feels dry naturally due to the fact that the texture (coil, kink, curl, or wave) of the hair strand makes it more difficult for the sebaceous oil glands in the scalp to release natural oils from root to ends. There are many types of conditioners. Good conditioners for afro-textured hair are deep and leave-in conditioners.

Moisturizing hair is a concept that is commonly misunderstood. Moisture comes from water. The ph balance of water should be 7, which is neutral, and allow the hair cuticles to lift and receive moisture. A good technique to use when applying moisture to hair is water, oil, and a sealant. The sealant is an emulsified product that helps to close the cuticles after moisture is received and protect the hair of chronic dryness from the air and any other elements.

Avoid ingredients such as chemicals, silicones, alcohols, mineral oil, and petroleum. They lead to unhealthy scalp and hair. Keeping the hair detangled can be a challenged, yet it could reap great benefits. It is important to always detangle hair gently and carefully, especially for afro-textured hair, which can suffer from hair breakage during this process. Detangling sections of hair from ends to roots will prevent tangles from piling on top of each other forming knots.

Low manipulation when caring for the hair can greatly minimize tangles.
To protect something means to keep it from harm or injury. So, how can hair become harmed or injured? This happens when hair becomes damaged. The following are some hair problems that can lead to damage: split ends, dryness, direct heat, harsh treatment, high manipulation, chemicals, etc.

Most hair has these problems, but if not placed under control it can become excessive and cause damaged or unhealthy hair. It is important to monitor how hair is cared for, and always use balance. A preventive measure to damaged hair is to wear a protective hairstyle. This requires all hair ends to be hidden. A low manipulation hairstyle does not keep-hidden hair ends yet requires less handling of your hair. It's also a good idea to sometimes cover the hair either with a hat, headdress, or scarf. Wear a satin bonnet to bed to minimize friction. Keep ends well preserved with trims and moisture.

SKIN

The primary cause of unhealthy skin is an unhealthy diet. There is naturally an only one skin type, which is called normal. Other skin types such as oily, dry, combination, and sometimes sensitive are schemes to appease our vanities with an intention to attract attention for business in the beauty market. If you really consider the skin on the body is not different from the skin on the face, such as skin on hand palms or feet soles. Yet the face *is* the place where most of the body's signs of impurities reflect itself. Eating a probiotic diet recommended in this book will eliminate the internal factors that could change normal skin.

In order to maintain healthy normal skin, there are some relevant things to be aware of and necessary actions to take. Pigmentation affects the integrity of the skin. It is a level of carbon found in human cells fixed by your genes and DNA. Some people have a greater concentration of pigment which aides as a protective barrier and gateway to better absorb vital nutrients.

A simple routine of cleansing, exfoliating, toning, moisturizing and protecting will grant well-preserved skin. Take proper care of all four poles of the body: face, feet, body, back (up, down, front, back). Cleansing the skin with water and a natural soap unclogs the pores from dirt, oils and toxins. Warm water opens the pores and after cleaning cool water closes the pores.

This should be done daily. Exfoliation deeply cleans the entire skin and texturizes it. This should be done regularly with a natural loofah or mask. It is optional to use a toner for the skin. It can be used two ways: as an astringent, or to refresh complexion by ridding grime.

It is important to use natural herbs, such as roses or witch hazel for this. It is not good to use alcohols or chemicals because this will unbalance the skins natural ph. Moisturize the skin daily to maintain hydration. This is done with water while natural butters, herbs, and oils will seal the moisture. Skin needs protection from many harsh things.

Environmental elements such as cold air and wind can be harsh to skin. It should be properly covered with thick 100% fabrics because the skin is a living organ that needs to 'breathe'. The sun can feel like a friend or an enemy to some depending on the pigment concentration. For instance, those with little to no skin pigmentation can receive adverse affects to the UV rays and need extra protection. Natural oils with SPF of at least 15 could provide protection for extended exposure to sunlight. Many studies have proven that those with a greater skin pigment concentration actually receive nutrients and other benefits from extended exposure to the sunlight. Most of all is mindfulness to have balance and gentle handling of your skin.

Some ladies and gentlemen may have reasons and preferences to pay special attention to the skin. For instance, eye creams; wrinkles, blemishes, stretch marks, and make-up are miscellaneous treatments for the skin. It's okay to do in moderation and using natural ingredients.

As for *sensitive skin types* usually the skin is simply reacting to an adverse ingredient that is not natural. All healthy normal skin should be sensitive to react towards anything adverse to it, such as chemicals. It is never good to put chemicals on the skin. A good rule to use when applying products to the skin is to question whether you can eat it. If you can't eat it, then you should not apply it to the skin because it eventually gets to the bloodstream just as the foods we eat. The following are some chemicals ingredients to avoid in products: Salicylic acid, talc, paraben, petrolatum, propylene glycol, fragrance, and boar bristles.

NAILS

The nails require very simple care to maintain quality health and beauty. Keep in mind that less is best. Basically, just as with hair nails should maintain a good balance of strength and moisture. Unhealthy nails provide signs for dysfunctions in the body systems. For instance, weak and brittle nails indicate an issue with the organs especially the liver. Also, each fingernail except the pinky should have a small crescent shape near the cuticles.

If this is not present then this is a sign of bad circulation. Healthy nails are the result of a healthy diet. From this point forward, the only necessity to support the nails is constant care. It is beneficial to have a regular regimen for both finger and toe nails to be cleansed, trimmed/filed/buffed, moisturized and protected.

Your finger and toenails become cleanse after a thorough bathe, and nails become especially cleanse after hand washing. Clean nails with soap and water and use a nailbrush to remove dirt under the nails. Trimming nails with clippers can help maintain strength especially when attempting to grow long nails. Filing nails helps to smooth and shape the nails. When filing do not use back and forth strokes that could lead to snags. Shape nails complementary to the cuticles with a wooden emery board. Buffing the nails supports stimulation of blood flow.

Moisturize nails with water and seal moisture with natural oils. Pay special attention to the cuticles. The cuticle layer should not be removed because it leaves the body viable to infection. Instead, push back the cuticles with an orangewood stick. Protect nails when using harsh chemicals, washing dishes, or gardening by wearing gloves or socks that are 100% fabrics or material.

Another form of protection is to not abuse them such as in biting or using them as tools. Sometimes special treatments can be given to the nails with extra cautions. If any nail has a fungus then this indicates that the body has an infection. Yet, this can be resolved with proper care for the body and herbs. Nail discoloration is a sign that the body's system is stressed. Use a sea salt and lemon mixture to exfoliate or remove discoloration from nails. Be careful when using nail polish and removers. Many polishes use harsh chemicals that could enter the bloodstream. Avoid these chemicals: formaldehyde, toluene, ethyl acetate, and camphor, Dibutyl Phthalate (DBP). It is better to use a water-based nail polish to paint nails. Prolonged use of nail polish could lead to yellow discoloration on the nails, which indicate that the system is toxic. When this happens stop polishing nails; detox the body; and resume the GLAD diet.

Why Natural?

The doctors, as I have stated prior are lying to you and trying to kill you. The food on the planet is the answer to our diseases, but we have to know what are the nutritional properties of the food that we are attempting to eat. It is a simple equation natural foods = complete mineral balance! Therefore if we follow this guide you will have a complete mineral balanced diet. Why is it so important that we have mineral balance in our diet? The answer is because the only substances that are important for our bodies to consume, are minerals. Here are the essential components to life:

As being called Human Beings we have forgotten what we are made of.

What is a Human Being? The word Hu-Man, comes from Humus Man. The Humus is the most perfect type of soil one can find. This humus soil is clay like, thick and formless but able to be formed. It is Jet Black and contains the seventeen essential minerals need to sustain life in a human body which are: Calcium, Zinc, Sulfur, Sodium, Selenium, Potassium, Molybdenum, Nickel, Phosphorus, Chloride, Cobalt, Copper, Fluorine, Iron, Manganese, Magnesium, Iodine. (Yisrael, 2011)

The ancient writings of truth (Holy Scriptures) constantly call us the sons of Adam or just Adam. What does Adam mean? Adam means; dirt-man, the true meaning of Hu-man is Humus Man, and Humus is the spongy like black soil in which the greatest concentration of the essential elements/minerals our body needs to survive.

Therefore let us look at this one scripture from Gen 2:7 And YAH Elohim formed man of the dust of the ground, and breathed into his nostrils the breath of life; and man became a living soul.

Here we see that the same components that made us become fully operational are the also the same components that will make sure were maintain health. The evidence is in the message of Gen. 1: 29. This is where the Most High let us know that all the food we should eat will be green food with the seed inside itself, and the fruit of the tree who's seed is inside itself. Furthermore, the Most High instructed his people to not sow our gardens, fields, or vineyards, with mingled seed. These instructions are very important to our health.

Natural green foods, and natural fruit contain high mineral contents that are absolutely essential for our bodies and green foods are compact with oxygen our body needs. What does oxygen do for our bodies besides give us air to breathe? Oxygen will kill any bacteria, virus, or infection in your body! If you do not have enough oxygen then all types of illness can live. Oxygen is also key to making sure our blood circulates, and our energy is hinged on the amount of oxygen we have.

Therefore a diet full of fresh, live green foods and an exceptional amount of water, will give us oxygen, aid our circulation and supply us with ample amounts of energy. These natural green foods are alkaline and will not produce acid, which will cause mucus to corrode your cells. Natural green foods are an excellent form of edible oxygen and a day should not pass without an abundant amount of green food.

The other great factors of natural fresh green foods are the minerals found in their roots, which are drawn from the natural rich soil the food should be growing in; by mingling the seeds of different plants you will start to deplete the soil of nutrients and cause the soil to be malnourished, and prone to drought . The fruit also contains a high mineral content. The minerals we are made of need to be constantly replenished from our diet. If we do not eat of the foods that contains the oxygen and minerals we are created from we will experience disease.

So what should a G.L.A.D. daily meal plan look like? Before we see what a meal plan should look like we must understand the correct times to eat our food.

"Woe to thee, O land, when thy king is a child, and thy princes eat in the morning! Blessed art thou, O land, when thy king is the son of nobles, and thy princes eat in due season, for strength, and not for drunkenness!" Ecc. 10:16-17

What does this mean? It means that always getting up in the morning and eating big fat pancakes, waffles, cheese eggs, 16oz cup of orange juice, four pieces of toast, steak , biscuits, bacon, ham, hash browns, pig brains, and whatever else we put on our plates; is definitely the wrong way to go! Our bodies operate on a rhythm, therefore we should attempt to follow the rhythm of nature and not create new song that is out of tune and off beat.

The rhythm I'm speaking of is the Circadian rhythm or Circadian clock. This is the natural cycle schedule of our bodies. By this rhythm is the best times to eat our food, have sex, exercise, sleep, study, etc. So what does our natural clock say is the best time to eat? From 12pm -7pm roughly. The reason is during the wee hours of the morning your body is assimilating foods and beginning to expel the waste from the prior day's meals. We have been taught to eat a large breakfast, and even larger lunch, and a gluttonous dinner. When in all actuality we should have a very small breakfast, and a light lunch and a hearty dinner, and none of this should be outside the specified time previously mentioned.

What does a light breakfast look like and when should I eat it? A light breakfast is water, and maybe a piece of fruit, like a plum, or a mineral shake, such as sea moss, or the Tamiym Super 7™ which provides all the essential minerals you would need to have to begin your day. This drink, or fruit should be eaten after you've drank your water, and began your day.

By lunch time you should eat a raw/Live meal, consisting of green leafy veggies, seeds and nuts (almonds, walnuts, brazil nuts), and of course water. Your last meal of the day should be your heaviest this is truly your first real meal and only meal of the day. This dinner; as it is called should be where we will consume our grains, blue or purple potatoes, Quinoa, Kammut, Wild, or Black Rice. It wouldn't hurt to throw in a nice salad at dinner time and always attempt to include sea veggies and of course water.

What about the snacks? Well, you want to be very careful about snacks. Today people call dollar menu items snacks, like two double cheese burgers. That's a very heavy meal. A snack is some nuts, a few pieces of dried fruit, or a piece of fruit or a smoothie, or some seeds. And not all at once either; one or the other! Now here comes the hard part! Treats! Candy, ice cream, cake, cinnamon buns, etc.

Just because you change your diet does not mean you will never enjoy anything sweet. The only difference is that we must know what is sweet and healthy and what is just down right poison. Refined food is poison so that means most of the treats you'll get from a store or restaurant will be poison.

There are Raw Pies, made from fruit and nuts (these are delicious!), and various fruits that are succulent! You can make vegan cakes and cookies like the recipe given earlier. And if you can afford it you can buy various treats made for the natural eater. As long as these dishes do not contain sugar and the other mentioned poisons, than every once in a while a treat will not hurt.

There are many ways to learn how to transition to a natural diet, and various classes given in different areas of the country to help you along with this process. Raw/Living food preparation courses are available, vegan cooking classes, vegan cook books, raw/living food recipe books, DVD'S and Health Seminars like the ones we do, which includes the book you are reading right now! We do not advocate one person or class over another, people have their preference on how they want to eat and live, we just urge that you consume natural foods, in order to have a happy, secure, healthy life!

Other ways to ensure a natural way of life is to make sure you have the right cooking and preparation equipment for the lifestyle change, and also have learn how to garden. The best food is the food you grow and raise yourself. Once you change the food that goes into your mouth it will have a chain reaction, you will begin to change the words that come out your mouth, and the environment will begin to represent the natural life you are living! You will become a proud and happy tree hugging Flower child of the Sun! Love will constantly be in the air and you will feel connected to the earth once again!

If you don't like living natural that is your preference but I guarantee if you try it, you will not leave it alone! Go on and give life a try!

Part 3: Home Herbalist 101

If you want to have a true revolution, then this means you will have to have a different social and political order of governance. In this case of Health, this means our reliance on the popular social order of health and wellness, would have to change. As we discussed in the first part of the book, Doctors, and those that work in the Allopathic or scientific field of

Health and Nutrition, are not healing or helping much of anything or anyone. Therefore it would be prudent for those attempting to return to a natural person they should discontinue from asking unnatural professionals to help you live.

The best way to ensure your health is well taken care of, is to do it yourself. Therefore we have developed a simple guide to helping you learn yourself and know what to do during various health crisis.

As the scriptures of Truth states in the Book of Ezekiel 47; *the fruit thereof shall be for meat, and the leaf thereof for medicine.*
If we want to be natural we have to follow the guidelines given by the maker of all!

Therefore the best way to deal with your health once you have to deal with a health crisis is to go to the herbs. We will show you 12 different Herb classifications and some herbs that fall under these classifications. The types of classifications are the most used amongst us today. The more you research you will find that there are an abundant of classifications for herbs.

After you've studied the different classifications and the corresponding herbs, you will be better equipped to know what kind of herb you might need to take for whatever ailment or issue you're attempting to heal. In addition to knowing the different categories of herbs/plants, it is also imperative to know the polarity of the nature. By this I mean it is important to understand how to treat ailments and various health issues depending on if they're acting in a male or female action or positive and negative, ying and yang...

In all things natural and even unnatural there is always positive and negative pole. For example if one is suffering from a mucus build up in their sinuses i.e. sinus infection. Then by the build happening indicates a female or negative action. Acid reflux is a male or positive action. Female is a nurturing, and slow moving, it builds and it grows; while male is fast, destructive, and hot.

Therefore to understand these actions are very important to healing yourself and using herbs. A so-called "heart attack" is not a fast or male action, actually a "heart attack" is a female action. Your heart will go in arrest or become under attack by the clogging of arteries, which build up over time until the point where your heart is no longer functioning correctly and you begin to undergo a cardiac arrest. Placing cayenne pepper under the tongue can stop an heart attack, or using a special formula that we carry called herbal adjustment by pure herbs ltd. These herbs are fast acting, and will cut or destroy build up i.e. mucus.

To maintain a clean bloodstream we must equip our homes with the correct foods to constantly clean our internal systems. Therefore if we eat with seasonings like various peppers, we will ensure a cleaning every time. Of course an excess of Cayenne pepper or others like it is not good, because as the properties of the herb indicates it will destroy. Therefore too much will destroy your esophagus lining, stomach lining and you will have a troublesome elimination process! Use discretion when using seasonings and make sure they are natural, fresh and organic.

Bread is another food that carries an obvious action- bread is made by a fermentation process this is obviously female. Bread rises, or builds, and this lets us know that bread, especially bread with yeast will be a female action in our bodies. Therefore if we do not want to suffer from various fungus related dis-eases e.g. yeast infections (Candidiasis), Thrush, eczema, sinus infections etc. then the eating of fermented products should not be consumed. As always, the moderation of a certain food is ok, breads made from spelt, rye, teff, quinoa, wild barley, kammut, and amaranth are good, esp. if they're unleavened breads. For anyone suffering a female dis-ease i.e. sinus, cold, cancer, fungal dis-eases should not consume bread, or anything fermented e.g. chocolate, cheese, and alcohol.

Our best method to preventing sickness in our homes is to maintain a clean environment, and this means a clean house, clean refrigerator, and clean body. A clean refrigerator should be of course clean from dirt, but also clean food. Clean food is food that is not defiled. Some clean foods are: Kale, Spinach, String Beans, Avocados, purple potatoes, zucchini squash, green lettuce, melons, seeded grapes, mangos, and more.

If you understand what I'm saying is; meat, eggs, milk, cheese, processed sugar, fish: shrimp, crabs, lobsters, krill, muscles, clams, oysters, calamari etc. are not clean foods. These foods should not enter into your house. Dead food brings and spreads a dead vibration within your energy field and will put a drag on your environment. Plus dead foods, will slowly kill you once you begin to consume them. Our healthiest way to eat is live natural foods.

What about emergency situations? Emergencies like: broken bones, cuts, heart attacks, seizures, strokes, burns, bleeding? As earlier mentioned Heart attacks, seizures, and strokes can all be stopped using Herbal Adjustment by Pure Herbs LTD.

Burns, Bruises, wounds, broken Bones, sprains, fractures, and other physical shock injuries can be assisted by using various topical herbs a few good ones are: Arnica, lobelia, St. Johns wart, Sangre De Grado (Dragon's Blood) Scarlet Brush, Aloes, Comfrey can be used but it is not a natural plant and therefore it should not be used internally and if you use it then do so by your own discretion externally.

A great thing for anyone wanting to rely on herbs for emergency healing would be to purchase an Herbal First aid Kit, or order the herbs from Tamiym Holistic Health ™ to make your own first aid kit. Poultices, Salves, Tinctures, Decoctions, Infusions, Macerations, and herbal baths are all various methods on how to heal urgent to very urgent conditions of all kind.

If muscle and skeletal repair is needed then using herbs externally will be ideal. A Salve, compress, or Poultice would be the best method. How to make any of these remedies is readily available on YouTube, and various Holistic Health books, and magazines. A Poultice is very easy to make and can help in numerous types of external problems.

For minor bruises a good poultice is Arnica and Lobelia: You can either use a mortar and pestle and grind the dried herbs into a powder or have the powder form and add enough water to where you make a paste, then place this on the effected area wrap it with plastic wrap and a ace bandage and leave on up to eight hours depending on the severity of the injury, it should be changed every 4-8 hours. Applying witch hazel after removing the poultice is good because witch hazel is an astringent and will close your pores, which were opened by the lobelia and arnica. This also shows the Male and female actions of the herbs

For internal emergencies liquid extracts of herbs are your best move. Herbs that have been extracted by water and alcohol or vegetable glycerin will quickly enter into your blood stream and immediately get to work. Therefore herbs that are stimulants like bee pollen, or ginseng can quickly restore ones vitality if they are in a extreme state of apathy.

Also for heart attacks a liquid extract of Capsicum (Cayenne Pepper) would be the best form to place under the tongue if the situation presents it self, or Herbal Adjustmen

12 Herb Classifications

ALTERATIVES

This is an herb or super-food that slows down the action of another herb being used as a curative. It puts everything back into harmony. Used according to the organ that needs it.

- Black Cohosh Root
- Cinnamon
- Mint

ANTIPERIODICS

This is an herb that breaks the cycle of periodic disharmonies in the body such as fevers, muscle spasms or headaches.

- Red Raspberry
- Vervain
- Feverfew

ANTI-INFLAMMATORY

It is used to reduce inflammations such as red, hot, swollen parts of the body from result of injury or infection. Garlic is a hybrid, acidic, fast- acting herb that breaks down substances without building up the body systems. A better alternative to garlic is bitter melon, which not only is fast- acting but also builds up the body systems.

- Cayenne
- Bitter Melon
- Slippery Elm
- Graviola

ANTI-SEPTICS

This herb destroys germs and disease-causing organisms and is nontoxic to cleanse wounds and prevent infections.

- Carasee
- Witch Hazel
- Guava Leaf

ASTRINGENTS

This herb caused contraction of blood vessels and body tissues, typically of the skin. It is good for use to reduce bleeding of minor abrasions. It can have a dry effect.

-
- Pau D' Arco
- Witch Hazel
- Tea Tree
- Rose

BITTER TONICS

An herb or super-food that gives a feeling of vigor or well being. It can also increase the appetite.

- Camu Camu
- Moringa
- Sea Moss (Irish Moss)
- Bladderwrack

CALMATIVES

These types of herbs have a sedative effect on the body. It relaxes your system and can be a good sleep aide.

- Passionflower
- Lavender
- Nettle
- Graviola

PURGATIVES

This herb or super- food is good for use to expel waste from the bowels.

- Graviola

- Bitter Melon
- Moringa

DIAPHORETICS

This type of herb induces perspiration for heavy sweating. It can aid the release of toxins from the system.

- Guaco
- aborandi Leaf
- Ginger

DIURETICS

This herb increases the passing of urine. It can be used as a mild detoxifier.

- Dandelion
- Guaco
- Cat's Claw

EXPECTORANTS

This herb promotes secretion of sputum by the air passages, especially used to treat coughs or colds.

- Mullein
- Guaco
- Cayenne
- Moringa

WOUND HEALER

These herbs are used to promote tissue formation and a scab.

- Shea Butter
- Bitter Melon
- Aloe Vera (topically only)
- Lobelia (Indian Tobacco) ,
- Arnica,

- Sangre De Grado
- Scarlet Brush

If you follow the advice give in this entire book, then you will be a home herbalist, or personal family healer. If you want to begin to help others, of course there are more in depth courses one can take or study with experienced naturopaths. There are schools popping up all over offering Master Herbalist Degrees, ND Degrees and more.

If you wish to take your search further on how to heal yourself and your family and community then more education would be suggested. We offer a launching pad to put you on the path to natural living and revolutionizing your life by returning to the natural state of being. The authors of this book operate Tamiym Holistic Health ™ and offer every herb mentioned in the book.

You can contact us by going to our website: www.blackplightnewsnet.com, or www.tamiyminc.com and if you are ever in the Atlanta, GA metro area you can visit us at the Natural Wholistic Health Village 1180 Ralph

David Abernathy Blvd. Atl, GA 30010. (404) 753-4555. We also offer various seminars to help you along the way to natural revolution. Call us at (513) 238-9482. Living natural is living healthy, being healthy naturally is freedom and peace, and let's all return to ourselves!

Bibliography

Wikipedia, 2011: The Human Genome Project
Http://www.wikipedia.com

YisraEL, IshYAH M. 2011. Escape From Babylon
IshYAH M. YisraEL: Decatur, GA

www.ingramcontent.com/pod-product-compliance
Lightning Source LLC
Chambersburg PA
CBHW050813290526
45792CB00001B/104